T0159008

Haitian Creole Medical Phrasebook
Presented in English, Creole, & Phonetics

Quick Creole
for
Medical
Personnel

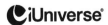

House of Hope Ministries, Inc.

Author: Dorothy Shumans

iUniverse

QUICK CREOLE FOR MEDICAL PERSONNEL
HAITIAN CREOLE MEDICAL PHRASEBOOK

iUniverse books may be ordered through booksellers or by contacting:

iUniverse
1663 Liberty Drive
Bloomington, IN 47403
www.iuniverse.com
1-800-Authors (1-800-288-4677)

ISBN: 978-1-5320-4121-1 (sc)
ISBN: 978-1-5320-4122-8 (e)

Library of Congress Control Number: 2018900805

Print information available on the last page.

iUniverse rev. date: 02/09/2018

<u>Other Books in the Hope Literature Series</u>

1. **Creole With A Smile** <u>*Kreyòl / English Dictionary*</u> – over 18,000 entries
2. **Creole With A Smile** <u>*Kreyòl / English Grammar Textbook*</u> with two CD's
3. **Levanjil / The Gospel** <u>in 6 Lessons</u> in Kreyòl and English, including **Songbook** with 20 songs & hymns in English and Kreyòl – all on **CD**

Contact Us

houseohope@yahoo.com

www.houseofhopemin.org

812-319-5972

House of Hope Ministries, Inc.
834 E. Main St.
Buffalo, Missouri 65622

Enndorsements

"We have found this dictionary to be superior to all others...". Tim Overholt, Christian Aid Ministries, Titayen, Haiti

"Your books are very detailed and I find them very useful." Lucia Van Maanen, missionary in Haiti

TABLE OF CONTENTS

T
A
B
L
E

O
F

C
O
N
T
E
N
T
S

QUICK CREOLE PRONUNCIATION GUIDE

In Creole, each symbol has one sound, except for the nasal combinations and dj, ch, tch and ou. Most consonants have the same sound as in English. **"pa"** before a verb indicates "negative", **"te"** = past tense, **"ap"** & **"pral"** = going to, and **"ta dwe"** = "have to".

NASAL SOUNDS

"on" like **"on"** as in "only" – bon, son, yon,

"an" like **"en"** as in "entrepreneur"

"en" like **"ai"** as in and "ain't"

OTHER SOUNDS & SPECIAL NOTES

"è" *pronounced like* **"e"** *as in* Eskimo

"e" *pronounced like* **"ay"** *as in* play, day, say

"i" *pronounced like* **"ee"** *as in* beet

"a" *pronounced like* **"a"** *as in* father

"ò" *pronounced like* **"o"** *as in* corn, born, horn

"o" *pronounced like* **"o"** *as in* home

"dj" *pronounced like* **"j"** *as in* jar

"ou" *pronounced like* **"oo"** *as in* boot

"ch" *pronounced like* **"ch"** *as in* Chicago

"tch" *pronounced like* "**tch**" *in* witch

"To do, make or create" can be translated **"fè". (feh).**

Meanings of "One"

One, *n.* *(counting number one)* – en
       (en, de, twa, kat, senk)
One, *pro. n.* *(one of my friends)* – youn
       (youn nan zanmi mwen)
One, *adj.* *(take one pill)* – yon
       (bwè yon grenn)

PRONUNCIATION GUIDE

PHONETIC PRONUNCIATION KEY / this book

ay – *sounds like*	**ā** – *as in c<u>a</u>ke*
eh – *sounds like*	**ĕ** – *as in <u>E</u>skimo*
ayh – *sounds like*	**<u>ai</u>** – *as in s<u>ai</u>nt and <u>ai</u>n't*
ee – *sounds like*	**<u>ee</u>** – *as in b<u>ee</u>t*
ah – *sounds like*	**<u>a</u>** – *as in f<u>a</u>ther*
oh – *sounds like*	**ō** – *as in <u>o</u>kra*
oo – *sounds like*	**<u>oo</u>** – *as in b<u>oo</u>t*
aw – *sounds like*	**<u>aw</u>** *in <u>aw</u>ful*
ohh – *sounds like*	**<u>o</u>** – *as in <u>o</u>nly*
	(nasal sound)
ahh – *sounds like*	**<u>en</u>** – *in <u>en</u>trepreneur*
	(nasal sound)
g – *sounds like*	**<u>g</u>** – *as in <u>g</u>oat*
j – *sounds like*	**<u>s</u>** – *as in mea<u>s</u>ure*
ng – *sounds like*	**<u>ng</u>** – *as in so<u>ng</u>*

ABDOMINAL DISORDERS

Have you had any pain?
Eske ou konn gen kèk doulè?
Ehs-keh oo **kohn** gayh **kehk doo-leh?**

Where?
Kikote?
Kee-koh-tay?

How long did it last?
Konbyen tan li te dire?
Koh-beey-ehn tah lee **teh** dee-ray?

Any cramps?
Ou gen kranp tou?
Oo gayh **krahmp** too?

Does it hurt when I press here?
Eske li fè ou mal lè m' peze la?
Ehs-keh lee **feh oo mahl** leh m' **pay-zay** lah?

Have you been vomiting?
Eske ou te vomi?
Ehs-keh oo **tay** voh-mee?

When?
Ki le?
Kee-leh?

Are your bowels moving every day?
Eske ou ap fè twalèt chak jou?
Ehs-keh oo ahp **feh twah-leht** shahk **joo?**

How many times a day?
Konbyen fwa chak jou?
Koh-beey-ehn fwah **shahk** joo?

Any blood in the urine / stools?
Lè ou ap pipi eske ou pa wè san?
Leh oo **ahp** peepee **ehs-keh** oo **pah** weh **sahh?**

Is it painful to urinate?
Eske li fè ou mal lè ou ap pipi?
ehs-keh lee **feh oo mahl** leh oo **ahp** pee-pee

We will need a stool sample.
N'ap bezwen yon zouti pou nou verifye sa.
Nahp behz-wayh yohh **zoo-tee** poo noo **vay-ree-feey-ay** sah.

ALLERGIES / ANAPHYLAXIS

Are you allergic to anything?
Eske ou gen alèji ak yon bagay?
Ehs-keh oo gayh **ahl-eh-jee** ahk yohh **bah-gahyee?**

Are you allergic to...?
Eske ou fè alèji ak ...?
Ehs-keh oo feh **ah-leh-jee** ahk...?

Penicillin?
Penisilin?
Peh-nee-see-leen?

Any medications?
Pyès medikaman?
Pee-yehs **may-dee-kah-mah**

Certain foods?
Kèk manje?
Kehk mahn-jay?

Were you stung by a bee?
Eske ou gen yon myèl ki te pike / mode ou?
Ehs-keh oo gehh yohh **meey-ehl** kee tay **pee-kay /**
moh-day oo?

Have you enhaled anything unusual?
Eske ou pa t' enspire kèk bagay ou pa t' konn abitye enspire?
Ehs-keh oo **pah t' ayn-spee-ray** kehk **bah-gahyee** oo **paht**
kohn ah-bee-tway ayn-spee-ray?

Have you ingested anything unusual?
Eske ou konn bwè / vale yon bagay ou pa t' konn pran?
Ehs-keh oo kohn **bweh / vah-lay** yohh bah-gahyee oo
pah t' kohn **prahn?**

Are you having abdominal pain?
Eske ou gen doulè nan vant ou?
Ehs-keh oo gehh **doo-leh** nah **vahnt** oo?

What?
Kisa?
Kee-sah?

Does your skin itch?
Eske po ou grate ou?
Ehs-keh poh oo **grah-tay oo?**

Do you have asthma?
Eske ou asmatik?
Ehs-keh oo
ahs-mah-teek?

ANATOMICAL & SYMPTOMATIC TERMS

Arm – *bra* / **brah**
Back – *do* / **doh**
Belly – *vant* / **vahnt**
Bladder – *blad* / **blahd**
Bleeding – *koule san* /
　　　koo-lay sahh
Blood – *san* / **sahh**
Breast – *sen* / **sayh / tay-tay**
Care for – *pran swen* /
　　　prah-swayh
Chest – *lestomak* / **lay-stoh-mahk**
Chills – *fredi* / **fray-dee**
Cold – *frèt* / **freht**
Constipated – *konstipe* /
　　　koh-stee-pay
Cut / injury – *blese* / **blay-say**
Diarrhea – *dyare* / **dee-ah-ray**
Ear – *zòrèy* / **zaw-ray**
Eye – *je* / **jay**
Eyelash – *plim je* / **pleem-jay**
Eyelid – *po je* / **poh-jay**
Esophagus – *esofaj* / **ay-soh-fahj**
Face – *figi* / **fee-gee**
Faranyx – *farenks* / **twoo-leh**
Fever – *fyèv* / **feey-ehv**
Finger – *dwèt* / **dweht**
Fingernail – *zong* / **zawng**
Foot – *pye* / **peey-ay**
Freckle – *tach* / **tahsh**
Gall bladder – *fyèl* / **feey-ehl**
Gut – *trip* / **treep**
Hand – *men* / **mayh**
Hair – *cheve* / **chay-vay**
Head – *tèt* / **teht**
Head ache - *tèt fè mal*
　　　teht feh mahl
Heal – *geri* / **gay-ree**
Heart – *kè* / **keh**

Hip – *anch* / **ahnsh**
Hot – *cho* / **shoh**
Infected – *enfekte* /
　　　ayh-fayk-tay
Inflammed – *anfle* / **ahh-flay**
Kidney – *renn* / **rayn**
Knee – *jenou* / **jay-noo**
Leg – *janm* / **jahm**
Lip – *po bouch* / **poh-boosh**
Liver – *fwa* / **fwah**
Lungs – *poumon* /
　　　poo-mohh
Mouth – *bouch* / **boosh**
Nose – *nen* / **nay**
Pain – *doulè* / **doo-leh**
Penis – *pijon* / *peni* /
　　　pee-johh / pay-nee
Pimple – *bouton* / **boo-tohh**
Rectum – *twou dèyè* /
　　　twoo day-yay
Seizure – *kriz* / **kreez**
Shoulder – *epòl* / **ay-pawl**
Sick – *malad* / **mah-lahd**
Skin – *po* / **poh**
Sore – *bouton* / **boo-tohh**
Stomach – *vant* / **vahnt**
Stomach ache – *vant fèh mal*
Swollen – *gonfle* / *gohh-flay*
Toe – *dwèt pye* /
　　　dweht-peey-ay
Toenail – *zong pye* / **zohng**...
Tongue – *lang* / **lahng**
Tooth – *dan* / **dahh**
Tooth ache – *dan fè mal*
Vagina – *vajin [bouboun]* /
　　　vah-jeen [boo-boon]
Voice box (laranyx) – *gòjèt*
　　　Gaw-jeht

6

APPOINTMENTS

Would you like to make an appointment?
Eske ou vle mete yon randevou?
Ehs-keh oo **vlay** may-tay yohh **rahn**-day-**voo?**

Which doctor do you want to see?
Ki doktè ou vle wè?
Kee dohk-**teh** oo **vlay** weh?

We have time available on (See days / months / numbers)
N'ap gen tan pou ou_____.
Nahp gehh **tahh** poo **oo_____.**

At ___. (See numbers & time)   Is that good for you?
A ___.ah   *Eske sa bon pou ou?*
                               Ehs-keh **sah** bohh **poo** oo?

What is your phone number?
Ki nimewo telefòn ou ye?
Kee nee-**may**-woh **tay**-lay-**fohn** oo yay?

Don't eat for ___ **(8 hours)** before the appointment.
Pa manje pou ___ (ywit è detan) avan randevou a.
Pah mahn-jay **poo** (yoo-eet eh day-tahh) **ah-vahh** rahn-day-voo **ah.**

TIME (See Days, Months, Seasons)

Tuesday, march 10th at 10:15.
Madi, dis Mas a dizè kenz. (day before month)
Mah-dee, dees mahs ah **dee**-zeh **kehnz**

8:00 o'clock	8:15 a.m.	8:30 a.m.
ywit è egzat	*ywit è kenz*	*ywit è trant*
yoo-eet **eh ehg**-zaht	**yoo**-eet **eh** kehnz	**yoo**-eet **eh** trahnt
8:45 a.m.	12:30 p.m.	1:00 p.m.
nev è mwen kenz	*midi trant*	*in è*
nehv eh **mway** kehnz	**mee**-dee **trahnt**	**een** eh
2:00 o'clock	12:00 o'clock	3:00 o'clock
dez è egzat	*midi egzat*	*twazè*
dayz eh **ayg**-zaht	**mee-dee** ayg-zaht	**twahz** eh

BASIC PHRASES / SMALL TALK

Good morning!
Bon jou!
<u>Boh</u> zhoo!

Good afternoon!
Bon swa!
<u>Boh</u> swah!

Good night!
Bon nwit!
<u>Boh</u> nweet!

Hello!
Alo!
<u>Ah</u>-loh!

How are you?
Komo ou ye?
<u>Koh-moh</u> oo yay?

Very well, thank you!
Tre byen, mèsi!
<u>Tray</u> bee-yehn <u>meh-see!</u>

Please.
Souple.
<u>Si-voo-play</u>

Thank you!
Mèsi!
<u>Meh-see!</u>

You're welcome!
Padekwa!
<u>Pa-day-kwah!</u>

Yes!
Wi!
<u>Wee!</u>

No!
Non!
<u>Noh!</u>

Pardon me!
Padone mwen!
<u>Pa-doh-nay</u> mway!

Good bye!
N'a wè!
<u>Nah</u> weh!

Mr.
Misye
<u>Mee</u>-see-ay

Mrs.
Madanm
<u>mah-dahm</u>

Miss
Madmwazèl
<u>mahd-mwah-zehl</u>

What is your name?
Kijan ou rele?
<u>Kee-zhahn</u> oo <u>ray-lay?</u>

My name is ...
Mwen rele ...
<u>Mwayh</u> ray-lay ...

Speak more slowly, please.
Pale pi dousman, sivouple.
<u>Pa-lay</u> pee <u>doos-mah</u>, see-voo-play.

At night
A nwit
<u>Ah</u> nweet

In the morning
Nan maten an
<u>nah</u> mah-<u>tay</u> ah

right here
isi
<u>ee</u>-see

BIRTH CONTROL

Do you use a birth control method?
Eske ou pran prekosyon pou ou pa asent?
Ehs-keh **oo** prahn **pray-koh-seey-ohh** poo **oo** pah **ah**-**saynt?**

Do you always use condoms during sex?
Eske ou toujou sèvi ak kapòt?
Ehs-keh oo **too-joo** seh-vee **ahk** kah-pawt?

Using condoms will also prevent sexually transmitted diseases.
Lè ou sèvi ak kapòt, sa k'ap anpeche maladi kontamine seksyalman.
Leh oo **seh-vee** ahk **kah-pawt,** sah **kahp** ahh-pay-shay **mahl-ah-dee** kohn-tah-mee-nay **sehk-see-yahl-mah.**

Do you take birth control pills?
Eske ou bwè grenn pou prekosyon ou pa ka asent?
Ehs-keh ou **bweh** grehn **poo** pray-koh-see-yohn **oo** pa **ah-saynt?**

Do you have a diaphragm?
Eske ou ap sèvi ak aparey ki rele diafram?
Ehs-keh oo **ahp** seh-vee **ahk** ah-pah-ray **kee** ray-lay **dee-ah-frahm?**

Would you like a prescription for birth control pills?
Eske ou vle preskripsyon grenn pou pran prekosyon ou pa asent?
Ehs-keh oo **vlay** yohh **pray-skreep-seey-ohh** grehn **poo** prahn **pray-koh-seey-ohh** oo **pah** ah-saynt?

BREATHING PROBLEMS

Are you having difficulty breathing?
Eske ou gen pwoblèm respirasyon?
Ehs-keh oo **gayh** pwoh-blehm **ray-spee-rah-seey-ohh**

With inspiration?
Ak enspirasyon?
Ahk ayhs-pee-rah-seey-ohh?

Expiration?
Ekspirasyon?
Ayks-pee-rah-
seey-ohh?

Did it come on suddenly?
Eske li parèt sou kò ou sibitman?
Ehs-keh lee pah-reht soo kaw oo
see-beet-mah?

Do you have pain?
Eske ou gen doulè?
Ehs-keh oo
gayh doo-leh

Has this happened before?
Eske sa te rive deja avan?
Ehs-keh sah **tay** ree-vay **day-jah** ah-vahh

When?
Kilè?
Kee-leh

Do you take any medications?
Eske ou te pran pyès medikaman?
Ehs-keh **oo** tay **prah** peey-ehs **may-dee-kah-mah**?

Which ones? Show me.
Kilès ladan yo? Montre m'.
Kee-lehs lah-dahn **yoh**? Moh-tray **m'**.

Do you have a cough?
Eske ou gen tous?
Ehs-keh oo **gayh** toos?

Does it produce sputum?
Eske l' fè ou krache?
Ehs-keh li **feh** oo **krah-shay**?

Any blood in the sputum?
Eske ou gen san nan krache a?
Ehs-keh oo **gayh** sahh **nah**
krah-shay?

Do you have...	tuberculosis?	Asthma?
Eske ou gen...	*tibèkiloz?*	*Asma?*
Ehs-keh oo gayh	tee-beh-kee-lohz	ahs-mah?

Emphysema?	Chronic bronchitis?
Anfezima?	*Bwonch kwonik?*
Ahh-fay-zee-mah?	Bwohsh kwoh-neek?

Do you have heart disease?
Eske ou gen kè fè mal?
Ehs-keh oo gayh keh feh mahl?

Do you have difficulty breathing at night?
Eske ou gen pwoblèm respire lannwit?
Ehs-keh oo gayh pwoh-blehm ray-spee-ray lah-nweet?

Do you breathe better sitting up?
Eske ou respire pi byen lè ou chita dwat?
Ehs-keh oo ray-spee-ray pee beey-ehn leh oo shee-tah dwaht?

Do you become short of breath during exertion?
Eske souf ou vin pi kout pandan ou ap fè egzèsyon? Spò?
Ehs-keh soof oo veen pee koot pah-dahh oo ahp feh ayg-zeh-see-yohh? (spaw)?

Did you inhale anything unusual?
Eske ou te enspire yon bagay ou pa t' konn abitye enspire?
Ehs-keh oo tay ayn-spee-ray yohh bah-gayee oo pah t' kohn ah-bee-tweh ayn-spee-ray?

Do you use an inhaler?	Do you smoke?
Eske ou sèvi ak yon inhelè?	*Eske ou fimen?*
Ehs-keh oo seh-vee ahk yohh	Ehs-keh oo fee-may?
een-hay-leh?	

BURNS

What caused the burn?
Kisa ki lakòz boule a?
Kee-sah kee **lah-kawz** boo-lay **ah**?

Hot water?   **Fire?**
Dlo cho?   *Dife?*
Dloh shoh?   **Dee-fay**?

Chemicals?
Chimi?
Shee-mee?

Electricity? (current)
Elektrisite? / (kouran)
Ay-layk-tree-see-tay? / **(koo-rah)**

Cover it.
Kouvri li.
Koo-vree **lee.**

Don't cover it.
Pa kouvri li.
Pah koo-vree **lee**.

Put cream / lotion
Mete krèm / losyon
May-tay krehm / **loh-see-yohh**

CALMING & COMFORTING PATIENT

You don't need to be afraid.
Ou pa bezwen pè.
Oo pah **behz-wayh** peh.

God is with us.
Bondye avèk nou.
Bohn-dee-ay ah-vehk **noo.**

He'll take good care of you.
L'ap pran swen ou byen.
Lahp prahh **swayh** ou **bee-yehn.**

He's the best doctor.
Li se pi bon dòktè pase tout lòt dòktè.
Lee say **pee** bohh **dohk-te** pah-say toot lawt **dohk-teh.**

He'll help you.
L'ap ede ou.
Lahp ay-day **oo.**

God is good. He knows everything. He's in control.
Bondye bon. Li Konnen tout bagay. Li gen tout pouvwa.
Bohn-dee-ay bohh. **Lee koh-nay** toot **bah-gahyee.**
Lee **gayh** toot **poov-wah.**

Pray for God to give you courage and strength.
Priye Bondye bay ou kouraj ak fòs.
Pree-ay **bohn-dee-ay** bah oo **koo-rahj** ahk **faws.**

Stay calm.
Rete trankil.
Ray-tay **trahng-keel.**

CHEST PAIN

Are you having chest pain?
Eske ou gen doulè nan lestomak?
Ehs-keh oo gayh doo-leh nahh stoh-mahk?

Where does it hurt?
Ki kote l' fè ou mal?
Kee koh-tay l' feh oo lay- Mahl?

When did it start?
Ki lè li te kòmanse?
Kee leh lee tay kaw-mah-say?

Is the pain severe?
Eske doulè a grav?
Ehs-keh doo-leh ah grahv?

Are you nauseated?
Eske ou gen kè plen?
Ehs-keh oo geh keh plehh

Does the pain radiate...
Eske doulè mache nan kò ou...?
Ehs-keh doo-leh mah-shay nahh kaw oo?

to the arms?
rive nan bra?
ree-vay nah brah?

to the back?
rive nan do?
ree-vay nah doh?

to the neck?
rive nan kou?
ree-vay nah koo?

Do you have a history of heart problems?
Eske ou konn gen pwoblem nan ke ou plizye fwa deja?
Ehs-keh oo gayh pwoh-blehm nah keh oo plee-zeey-ay fwah day-jah?

Have you ever had a heart attack?
Eske ou konn gen atak kè?
Ehs-keh oo kohn gayh ah-tahk keh?

Do you have high blood pressure?
Eske ou gen tansyon wo? Eske ou fè tansyon?
Ehs-keh oo gayh tah-seey-ohh woh? Ehs-keh oo feh tah-seey-ohh?

This will help the pain.
Sa kapab soulaje doulè a.
Sah kah-pahb soo-lah-jay doo-leh ah.

C
H
E
S
T

P
A
I
N

14

CLEAN CATCH INSTRUCTIONS
(To Copy & Post)

Use this antiseptic towelette to cleanse the external genitalia / the head of the penis.

1. *Itilize sèvyèt ijenik sa a pou ou pwòpte deyò bouboun ou / tèt pijon ou.*

Allow the initial portion of the urine stream to escape.

2. *Pèmèt premye ti gout pipi a ale.*

Collect the mid-portion of the urine stream in the container.

3. *Mete pwochèn pòsyon pipi a ki pwòp nan veso a.*

C
L
E
A
N

C
A
T
C
H

I
N
S
T
R
U
C
T
I
O
N
S

DAYS, MONTHS & SEASONS

Monday	Tuesday	Wednesday	Thursday
Lendi	*Madi*	*Mèkredi*	*Jedi*
lehn-dee	**mah**-dee	**meh**-kray-**dee**	**Jay**-dee

Friday	Saturday	Sunday
Vandredi	*Samdi*	*Dimanch*
vahn-dray-**dee**	**sahm**-dee	**dee-**mahsh

January	February	March
Janviye	*Fevriye*	*Mas*
jahh-vee-**ay**	**fay**-vree-**ay**	**mas**

April	May	June
Avril	*Me*	*Jen*
ah-vreel	**may**	**jayh**

July	August	September
Jiye	*Out*	*Septanm*
jee-ay	**oot**	**sayp**-tahm

October	November	December
Oktòb	*Novanm*	*Desanm*
ohk-tawb	**noh**-vahm	**day**-sahm

Spring	Summer	Fall	Winter
Prentan	*Ete*	*Otòn*	*Ivè*
prayh-tahh	**ay**-tay	**oh**-tawn	**ee**-veh

DEPRESSION, ANXIETY SCREENING

Have you been feeling sad or empty?
Eske ou konn santi ou tris oubyen vid?
<u>Ehs-keh</u> oo <u>kohn</u> sahn-tee <u>oo</u> trees <u>oo-beey-ehn</u> veed?

Does your sadness cause problems in your life?
Eske tristès la kòz pwoblèm nan lavi ou?
<u>Ehs-keh</u> trees-tehs <u>lah</u> bahee <u>lah-vee</u> oo <u>pwoh-blehm</u>?

Do you find pleasure in daily activities?
Eske ou pran plezi nan aktivite ou fè chak jou?
<u>Ehs-keh</u> oo <u>prah</u> play-zee <u>nah</u> ahk-tee-vee-te <u>oo</u> feh <u>shahk</u> <u>Joo?</u>

Do you often sleep during the day?
Eske ou konn domi lajounen souvan?
<u>Ehs-keh</u> oo kohn <u>doh-mee</u> lah-joo-nayh <u>soo-vahh?</u>

Do you ever have thoughts of suicide?
Eske ou konn fè move panse pou ou touye tèt ou?
<u>Ehs-keh</u> oo <u>kohn</u> feh <u>moh-vay</u> pahh-say <u>poo</u> oo <u>too-yay</u> teht <u>oo?</u>

Are you often afraid or anxious?
Eske ou konn pè oubyen nève souvan?
<u>Ehs-keh</u> oo <u>kohn</u> peh <u>oo-beey-ehn</u> neh-vay <u>soo-vahh?</u>

Do you have trouble sleeping at night?
Eske ou gen pwoblèm pou ou domi lannwit?
<u>Ehs-keh</u> oo gayh <u>pwoh-blehm</u> poo <u>oo</u> doh-mee <u>lah-nweet?</u>

I will write a prescription for you.
M'ap ekri yon preskripsyon pou ou.
<u>Mahp</u> <u>eh-kree</u> yohh <u>pray-skreep-seey-ohh</u> poo <u>oo.</u>

The medication may take several weeks to be effective.
Medikama saa ap pran kèk semèn pou l' fè efè sou ou.
<u>May-dee-kah-mah</u> sah-ah <u>ahp prahn</u> kehk <u>say-mehn</u> poo l' feh <u>ay-feh</u> soo <u>oo.</u>

DIABETES

Are you a diabetic?
Eske ou gen sik? Eske ou fè sik?
Ehs-keh oo **gayh seek**? Ehs-keh oo **feh seek**?

Do you take insulin?
Eske ou pran ensilin nan?
Ehs-keh oo prah **ehn-see-lehn?**

with each meal?
ak chak manje?
ahk shahk **mahn-jay?**

What type? (kind)
Ki kalite?
Kee **kah-lee-tay?**

oral or by injection?
nan bouch oubyen pa piki?
nah boosh **oo-bee-yehn** pah
pee-kee?

When did you last take insulin?
Ki dènye fwa ou te pran insilin nan?
Kee **dehn-yay** fwah **oo** tay **prahn** ehn-see-lehn?

Do you self-test for blood sugar?
Eske ou te fè egzamen pou sik la oumenm?
Ehs-keh oo **feh** ayg-zah-may **poo** seek **lah** oo-mehm?

Have you been taking insulin on a regular basis?
Eske ou abitwe pou pran ensilin nòmalman?
Ehs-keh oo **ah-bee-tweh** poo **prahn** ehn-see-lehn
naw-mahl-mah?

When did you eat last?
Ki dènye fwa ou te manje?
Kee **dehn-yay** fwah oo **tay** mahn-jay?

Do you have a special diet?
Eske ou gen yon fason ou kontwole manje ou?
Ehs-keh oo **gayh** yohh **fah-soh** oo **kohn-twoh-lay** mahn-jeh **oo?**

Have you been ill lately / recently?
Eske ou pa gen twò lontan depi ou te malad?
Ehs-keh oo **pah** gayh **twaw** lohn-tah **deh-pee** oo **tay** mah-lahd?

D
I
A
B
E
T
E
S

Have you been tested for the H.I.V. virus?
Eske ou te pran tès SIDA deja?
Ehs-keh oo tay prahn tehs see-dah deh-jah?

Have you ever injected drugs with a needle?
Eske ou konn mete dwòg nan san ou?
Ehs-keh oo kohn may-tay dwawg nah sahh oo?

We suggest you have a blood test for H.I.V. virus.
Nou sijere ou fè yon tès pou SIDA.
Nou see-jay-ray ou feh yohh tehs poo see-dah.

The blood test was negative (positive) for H.I.V.
Rezilta tès SIDA a te negatif / positif.
Ray-zeel-tah tehs see-dah-ah tay neh-gah-teef / poh-zee-teef.

We suggest another test in three months.
Nou mande ou pou ou pran yon lòt tès apre 3 mwa.
Noo mahn-day oo poo oo prahn yohh lawt tehs ah-pray twah mwah.

IMMUNIZATIONS

Has your child received any immunizations?
Eske pitit ou a te pran kèk vaksen?
<u>Ehs-keh</u> pee-teet <u>oo ah</u> tay <u>prahh</u> kehk <u>vahk-sayh</u>?

Do you know which immunizations?   **When?**
Eske ou konnen ki kalite piki?   *Kilè?*
<u>Ehs-keh</u> oo <u>koh-nay</u> kee <u>kahl-ee-tay</u> pee-kee?   <u>Kee-leh?</u>

Do you have an immunization card?
Eske ou gen yon kat ki montre m' ki piki li gen?
<u>Ehs-keh oo gayh yoh kaht</u> kee <u>mohn-traym</u> kee <u>pee-kee</u> lee <u>gayh?</u>

When was your last tetanus booster vaccination?
Ki lè dènye fwa ou te pran vaksen pou tetanous?
<u>Kee leh</u> dehn-yay <u>fwah</u> oo <u>tay</u> prahh <u>vahk-sayh</u> poo <u>teh-tah-noos?</u>

You need a tetanus booster vaccination.
Ou bezwen yon vaksen pou tetanous.
<u>Oo behz-wayh</u> yohh <u>vahk-sayh</u> poo <u>teh-tah-nous.</u>

If you are over 65, you should have an influenza vaccination every year in the autumn and pneumococcal every 5 years.

Si ou gen plis pase 65 lane, ou dwe pran yon vaksen inflouenza chak ane nan sezon lotonn e noumoni chak senk lane.

<u>See</u> oo <u>gayh</u> plees <u>pah-say</u> swah-sahn-kehnz <u>lah-nay</u>, oo <u>dway</u> prahn <u>yohh</u> vahk-sayh <u>een-floo-ehn-zah</u> shak <u>lah-nehh</u> nah <u>say-zoh</u> loh-tohn e noo-moh-nee <u>shak</u> sehnk <u>lah-nay.</u>

Please inform us of any bad reactions such as fever, crying, or seizures following any vaccination,

Souple, mete nou okouran si piki a fè move efè tankou fyèv, rele, oubyen kriz.

Soo-play, <u>may-tay</u> noo <u>oh-koo-rahh</u> see <u>pee-kee</u> ah feh moh-vayh <u>ay-feh</u> tahn-koo <u>feey-ehv</u>, ray-lay, <u>oo-beey-ehn</u> kreez.

IMMUNIZATIONS

Copy and post this information.
Basic Information for Vaccinations

The DTP vaccine (Diptheria, Tetanus, & Pertussis) should be given at age 2 months, 4 months, 6 months, and at 5 years of age.

Vaksen DTP a bon pou timoun 2 mwa, 4 mwa, 6 mwa, epi rive nan 5 lane.

The MMR vaccine (Measles, Mumps, & Rubella) should be given at age 15 months and again at age 5 years.

Vaksen MMR bon pou timoun 15 mwa epi tou ankò ak sa yo ki gen 5 lane.

The Hib (Influenza) vaccine should be given at 2 months, 4 months, 6 months, and 15 months of age.

Vaksen Hib (Influenza) ou dwe bay timoun ki gen 2 mwa, 4 mwa, 6 mwa, epi 15 mwa.

The Hepatitis B vaccine is recommended at birth, at 2 months, and at 6 months of age.

Vaksen Epatit B a rekomande pou timoun ki fenk fèt, ki gen 2 mwa, epi ki gen 6 mwa.

The OPV vaccine (Polio) should be given at 2 months, 4 months, 12 months, & at 5 years of age.

Vaksen OPV (Polio) a ou dwe bay timoun ki gen 2 mwa, 4 mwa, 12 mwa, ak 5 lane.

I
M
M
U
N
I
Z
A
T
I
O
N
S

INJECTIONS & MEDS

I'm going to give you an injection.
Mwen pral ba ou yon piki.
<u>Mwayh</u> **<u>prahl bah oo</u>** yohh **<u>pee-kee</u>**.

Turn on your side.	Relax!
Vire sou bò ou.	*Kalme! Relaks!*
<u>Vee-ray</u> soo **<u>baw oo</u>**.	**<u>Kahl-may!</u>** Ray-lahks!

I am placing this intravenous needle in your arm.
M'ap mete piki pou venn sa a nan bra ou.
<u>Mahp</u> may-tay **<u>pee-kee poo vayn sah-ah</u>** nah **<u>brah</u>** oo.

Squeeze your fist.	Like this!
Fè pwen ak men ou.	*Konsa!*
<u>Feh pwayh</u> ahk mayh oo.	**<u>Kohn-sah!</u>**

Keep your arm straight.	It will sting for a moment.
Kenbe bra ou dwat.	*L'ap boule ou pou yon ti moman.*
<u>Kaym-bay</u> brah oo **<u>dwaht</u>**.	Lahp **<u>boo-lay oo</u>** **<u>poo</u>** yoh **<u>tee</u>** moh-mah.

The apparatus will stay in your arm.
Aparey a ap rete nan bra ou.
<u>Ah-pah-ray</u> ah **<u>ahp</u>** ray-tay **<u>nahh</u>** brah **<u>oo.</u>**

Be careful not to pull the apparatus out.
Fè atansyon pou ou pa retire aparey nan bra ou.
<u>Feh</u> ah-tah-seey-ohh **<u>poo oo</u>** pah **<u>ray-tee-ray</u>**
ah-pah-ray **<u>nah</u>** brah **<u>oo</u>**.

I have <u>a / some</u> pills for you to take.
Mwen gen <u>yon / kèk</u> grenn pou m' bay ou.
<u>Mway gayh</u> yohh / kehk grehn **<u>poo-m</u>** bah **<u>oo.</u>**

Very Important!	*Trèz enpòtan!*	**<u>Trehz ayh-paw-tahh!</u>**

Take ____ pill(s) ____times a day until they are all gone. (See numbers)
Bwè ____ grenn ____ fwa chak jou jiskaske yo fini.
<u>Bweh</u> ____ <u>grehn</u> ____ fwah shahk joo **<u>jees-kahs-keh</u>** yoh **<u>fee-nee</u>**.

Remove your bra, please.
Retire soutyen ou, sivouple.
<u>Ray-tee-ray</u> soo-tee-yehh oo **see-voo-play**.

I will place your breast on this plate (shelf).
M'ap mete tete ou sou etaj sa.
<u>Mahp</u> may-tay **tay-tay oo** soo **ay-tahj** sa.

The machine will squeeze your breast.
Aparey sa a pral peze tete ou.
<u>Ah-pah-ray</u> sah-ah **prahl** pay-zay **tay-tay oo**.

The squeezing may feel uncomfortable.
Ou ka santi ou pa alèz.
Oo kah **sahn-tee** oo **pah ah-lehz**.

Stand here.
Kanpe la.
<u>Kahm-pay</u> lah.

MEDICAL ASSESSMENT

Do you have pain?
Eske ou gen doulè?
Ehs-keh oo **gayh doo-leh?**

Where does it hurt?
Ki kote l' fè mal?
Kee koh-tay l' **feh** ou **mahl?**

Do you have...
Eske ou gen...
Ehs-keh oo gayh...

diabetes?
(fè) sik?
(feh) seek

Heart problems?
Pwoblèm nan kè?
Pwoh-blehm nah keh?

Allergies?
Alèji?
Ah-leh-jee?

Lung problems?
Pwoblèm nan poumo?
Pwoh-blehm nahh **poo-moh?**

Any blood in the urine?
Eske ou wè san nan pipi?
Ehs-keh oo **weh** sahn nah pee-pee?

Are you moving your bowels normally?
Eske ou ap fè dijesyon nòmalman?
Ehs-keh oo **ahp** feh **dee-jeh-seey-ohn** naw-mahl-mah?

Do you have diarrhea?
Eske ou ap fè dyare?
Ehs-keh oo **ahp** feh **dee-ah-ray?**

Any blood in the stools?
Eske ou wè matye nan twalèt ou?
Ehs-keh oo weh **mah-tee-ay** nah twah-leht oo?

Does it hurt when I press here?
Eske ou santi doulè lè m' touche ou isi?
Ehs-keh oo **sahn-tee** m' too-chay oo ee-see?

How long have you been ill?
Depi konbyen tan ou malad?
Day-pee **kohh-bee-yehn tahn** oo **mah-lahd?**

Have you ingested anything unusual?
Eske ou te vale kèk bagay ou pa abitwe vale?
Ehs-keh oo **tay** vah-lay **kehk** bah-gahy-ee **oo** pah
ah-bee-tway vah-lay?

Has this ever happened before?
Eske sa konn rive ou deja?
Ehs-keh sah **kohn** ree-vay **oo?**
day-jah?

Relax!
Kalme!
Kahl-may!

Permit me....
Pèmèt mwen....
Peh-meht mwayh

Cough!
Touse!
Too-say

Again!
Ankò!
Ahng-kaw!

Lean forward, please.
Bese devan, sivouple.
Bay-say day-vahh, **see-voo-play.**

Inhale.
Enspire.
Ayn-spee-ray,

Exhale.
Ekspire.
Ayks-pee-ray.

Breathe deeply.
Respire fò.
Ray-spee-ray faw.

Are you having difficulty breathing?
Eske ou gen pwoblèm pou ou respire?
Ehs-keh oo gayh pwo-blehm **poo** oo **ray-spee-ray?**

With inspiration?
Lè ou enspire?
Leh oo ayn-spee-ray?

With expiration?
Lè ou ekspire?
leh oo ehks-pee-ray?

Do you have a cough?
Eske ou gen tous?
<u>Ehs-keh</u> oo gayh <u>toos?</u>

Does it produce sputum?
Eske l' fè ou krache?
<u>Ehs-keh l'</u> feh oo <u>krah-shay?</u>

Do you have ...?
Eske ou gen...?
<u>Ehs-keh oo gayh...?</u>

Chronic bronchitis?
Bwonch kwonik?
<u>Bwohsh kwoh-neek?</u>

Asthma?
Asma?
<u>Ahs-mah?</u>

Emphysema?
Enfasima?
<u>Ayh-fah-see-mah?</u>

Do you smoke?
Eske ou fimen?
<u>Ehs-keh oo fee-may?</u>

Do you have epilepsy?
Eske ou gen kriz / epilepsy?
<u>Ehs-keh oo gayh</u> kreez / ay-pee-layp-see?

What medicines do you take?
Ki medikama ou ap pran?
<u>Kee</u> may-dee-kah-mah <u>oo</u> ahp <u>prahn?</u>

Are you pregnant?
Eske ou ansent?
<u>Ehs-keh oo</u> <u>ahh-saynt?</u>

How many months?
Konbyen mwa ou genyen?
<u>Kohh-beey-ehn</u> mwah oo
<u>gayh-yayh?</u>

Are you allergic to any medications?
Eske ou gen alèji ak kèk medikaman?
<u>Ehs-keh oo gayh</u> <u>ah-leh-jee</u> ahk kehk <u>may-dee-kah-mah?</u>

Are you having chest pains?
Eske ou gen lestomak fè mal?
<u>Ehs-keh</u> oo gayh <u>lay-stoh-mahk</u> feh <u>mahl?</u>

Did the pain occur suddenly?
Eske doulè a te parèt britsoukou?
Ehs-keh **doo-leh ah** tay pah-reht **breet-soo-koo?**

Point to the pain.
Montre m' kote l' fè ou mal.
Moh-traym **koh-tay l'** feh oo mahl?

Are you nauseated?
Eske ou gen kè plen?
Ehs-keh oo gayh **keh playh?**

Are you a diabetic?
Eske ou fè sik?
Ehs-keh oo **feh seek?**

Do you take insulin?
Eske ou pran ensilin?
Ehs-keh oo prahn **ayh-see-leen?**

Oral or by injection?
Pa bouch oubyen pa piki?
Pah boosh **oo-bee-yehn** pah **pee-kee?**

When did you last take insulin?
Ki dènye fwa ou te pran ensilin?
Kee **dehn-yay fwah** oo **tay** prahn **ayh-see-leen?**

Can you feel my touch?
Eske ou santi m' touche ou?
Ehs-keh oo **sahn-tee-m'** too-shay **oo?**

Have this prescription filled.
Al ranpli preskripsyon sa a.
Ahl rahm-plee **pray-skreep-see-yohh** sah ah?

NEUROLOGICAL DISORDERS

Do you have a headache?
Eske ou gen tèt fè mal?
<u>Ehs-keh</u> oo gayh <u>teht feh mahl?</u>

Are you dizzy?
Eske ou gen tèt vire?
<u>Ehs-keh</u> oo gayh <u>teht vee-ray?</u>

Are you nauseated?
Eske ou gen kè plen?
<u>Ehs-keh</u> oo gayh <u>keh plehh?</u>

When did the symptoms begin?
Depi kilè sentom nan kòmanse?
<u>Day-pee</u> kee-leh <u>sehn-tawm</u> nah <u>kaw-mahn-say?</u>

Do you have a history of headaches / epilepsy?
Eske ou abitwe gen tèt fè mal / kriz?
<u>Ehs-keh</u> oo <u>ah-bee-tweh</u> gayh <u>teht feh mahl</u> / kreez?

What day is this?
Jodia se ki jou?
<u>Joh-dee-ah</u> say <u>kee</u> joo?

What month is this?
Nan ki mwa nou ye?
Nahh <u>kee</u> mwah <u>noo</u> yay?

Can you feel my touch?
Eske ou kapab santi mwen touche ou?
<u>Ehs-keh</u> oo <u>kah-pahb sahn-ti</u> mway <u>too-shay oo?</u>

Does it feel sharp or dull?
Eske ou santi l' piki piki oubyen ou santi l' toupiti.
<u>Ehs-keh</u> oo <u>sahn-tee</u> l' pee-kee pee-kee, <u>oo-bee-yehn</u> sahn-tee l' <u>too-pee-tee?</u>

Squeeze my fingers!
Peze dwèt mwen!
<u>Pay-zay</u> dweht mwayh?

Move your arm / legs!
Jwe ponyèt ou / pye ou!
<u>Jway</u> pohh-yeht <u>oo</u> / <u>pee-ay</u> oo?

NUMBERS

English	Kreyòl	Phonetics
0	zero	*zewo*	**zay**-who
1	one	*en*	**ayh**
2	two	*de*	**day**
3	three	*twa*	**twah**
4	four	*kat*	**kaht**
5	five	*senk*	**sayhnk**
6	six	*sis*	**sees**
7	seven	*sèt*	**seht**
8	eight	*ywit*	**y**weet
9	nine	*nèf*	**nehf**
10	ten	*dis*	**dees**
11	eleven	*onz*	**ohnz**
12	twelve	*douz*	**dooz**
13	thirteen	*trèz*	**trehz**
14	fourteen	*katoz*	**kah**-tohz
15	fifteen	*kenz*	**kehnz**
16	sixteen	*sèz*	**sehz**
17	seventeen	*disèt*	**dee**-seht
18	eighteen	*dizywit*	**deez**-yweet
19	nineteen	*diznèf*	**deez**-nehf
20	twenty	*ven*	**vehh**
21	twenty-one	*vente-en*	**vehn**-tay-**ayh**
22	twenty-two	*venn-de*	**vehn**-day
30	thirty	*trant*	**trahnt**
31	thirty-one	*trante-en*	**trahn**-tay-**ayh**
32	thirty-two	*trann-de*	**trahn**-day
40	forty	*karant*	**kah**-rahnt
41	fourty-one	*karante-en*	**kah**-rahn-**tay**-ayh
42	forty-two	*karann-de*	**kah**-rahn-**day**
50	fifty	*senkant*	**sehng**-kahnt
51	fifty-one	*senkante-en*	**sehng**-kahn-**tay**-ayh
52	fifty-two	*senkann-de*	**sehng**-kahn-**day**
60	sixty	swasant	swah-sahnt
61	sixty-one	*swasante-en*	**swah**-sahn-**tay**-ayh
62	sixty-two	*swasann-de*	**swah**-sahn-**day**
70	seventy	*swasann-dis*	**swah**-sahn-**dees**
71	seventy-one	*swasant-onz*	**swah**-sahnt-**ohnz**
72	seventy-two	*swasann-douz*	**swah**-sahn-**dooz**
80	eighty	*katreven*	**kah**-tray-**vehh**
81	eighty-one	*katreven-en*	**kah**-tray-**vehn**-ayh
90	ninety	*katrevenn-dis*	**kah-tray-vehn**-dis
91	ninety-one	*katreven-onz*	**kah-tray-vehn-onz**
100	one-humdred	*san`*	**sahh**

OB / GYN

When was your last menstruation?
Ki dènye fwa ou te gen règ ou?
<u>Kee</u> dehn-yay <u>fwah oo tay</u> gayh <u>rehg</u> oo?

Is this your first childbirth?
Eske sa se premye akouchman ou?
<u>Ehs-keh</u> sa say <u>pray-meey-ay</u> ah-koosh-mah <u>oo?</u>

Have you had problems with previous pregnancies?
Eske ou janm gen pwoblèm avèk lòt akouchman?
<u>Ehs-keh</u> oo <u>jahm</u> gayh <u>pwoh-blehm</u> ah-vehk <u>lawt</u>
ah-koosh-mah?

The birth may need to be cesarean.
Akouchman saa mande sezaryèn.
<u>Ah-koosh-mah</u> sah-ah <u>mahn-day</u> say-zah-reey-ehn.

Has your water broken?
Eske ou te kase lezo?
<u>Ehs-keh</u> oo <u>tay</u> kah-say
<u>lay-zoh</u>?

Are you havingconractions?
Eske ou santi kontraksyon?
<u>Ehs-keh</u> oo <u>sahn-tee</u>
kohn-trahk-seey-ohh?

Do you need pain relief?
Eske ou bezwen yon bagay ki pou soulaje doulè a?
<u>Ehs-keh</u> oo behz-wen <u>yohh bah-gahyee</u> kee poo <u>soo-lah-jay</u>
doo-leh <u>ah?</u>

You may (<u>not</u>) walk around.
Ou kapab fè yon ti mache / ou <u>pa ta</u> dwe mache.
Oo <u>kah-pahb</u> feh <u>yoh</u> tee <u>mah-shay</u> / oo <u>pah tah dway</u>
mah-shay.

Push during the contraction.
Pouse pandan kontraksyon an.
<u>Poo-say pah-dah</u>
<u>kohn-trahk-seey-ohh</u> an.

Don't push!
Pa pouse!
<u>Pah</u> poo-say!

Breathe!
Respire!
<u>reh-spee- ray</u>

It's a boy / girl!
Se yon gason / yon fi!
<u>Say</u> yohh <u>gah-sohh</u> / yohh <u>fee!</u>

He's/she's beautiful!
Li bèl!
<u>Lee</u> behll!

Are you pregnant?
Eske ou ansent?
<u>Ehs-keh</u> oo <u>ah-saynt?</u>

We need a urine specimen.
Nou bezwen pran pipi.
Noo <u>behz-wayh</u> prahn <u>pee-pee.</u>

Is it painful to urinate?
Eske l' fè ou mal lè ou ap pipi?
Ehs-keh l' <u>feh</u> oo <u>mahl</u> leh <u>oo</u> ahp <u>pee-pee?</u>

Do you have a vaginal discharge?
Eske ou gen dechay parèt nan kilòt ou?
<u>Ehs-keh</u> oo gayh <u>day-chahyee</u> pah-reht <u>nah</u> kee-lawt <u>oo?</u>

We need to take a cervical tissue sample.
Nou bezwen fè egzamen pou pran echantiyon tisi sèviks.
Noo behz-wehh <u>feh ayg-zah-may</u> poo prahn
<u>ay-shah-teey-ohh</u> tee-see <u>seh-veeks.</u>

I am going to insert the speculum.
Mwen pral antre spekilom nan.
Mwayh <u>prahl</u> ahn-tray <u>speh-kee-lawm</u> nah

Diaphram?
Dyafram?
<u>dee-ah-frahm?</u>

It may feel cool.
Ou ka santi l' fre.
Oo kah <u>sahn-tee</u> l' fray

Condom?
Kapòt?
<u>Kah-pawt?</u>

Are you currently sexually active?
Eske ou toujou fe bagay?
Ehs-keh oo too-joo **feh bah-gahyee**

Pill? **Shot?**
Grenn? *Piki?*
<u>grehn?</u> <u>pee-kee</u>

Do you use a birth control method?
Eske ou sèvi ak yon metod pou kontwole akouchman?
Ehs-keh oo <u>seh-vee</u> ahk yohh <u>may-tawd</u> poo <u>koh-twohl-ay</u>
<u>ah-koosh-mah?</u>

PATIENT COMPLAINTS

I am ____.
Mwen____/.
Mwayh   .

I am weak.
Mwen fèb.
Mwayh fehb.

I am ill.
Mwen malad.
Mwayh mah-lahd.

I am bleeding.
M'ap koule san.
Mahp koo-lay sahh.

I am dizzy.
Mwen gen vètij / tèt vire.
Mwayh gayh veh-teej / teht vee-ray.

I'm constipated.
Mwen konstipe.
Mwayh kohh-stee-pay.

I am hot / cold.
Mwen cho / frèt.
Mwayh shoh / freht.

I am pregnant.
Mwen ansent.
Mwayh ah-saynt.

I have been raped.
M' te pran sizo.
M' tay prahn see-zoh.

It is painful to urinate.
Li fè m' mal lè m'ap pipi.
Lee feh m' mahl leh mahp pee-pee.

I have tuberculosis / emphysema / asthma.
Mwen gen tibèkiloz / enfazima / asma.
Mwayh gayh tee-beh-kee-lohz / ayh-fah-zee-mah / ahs-mah.

My lungs are congested.
Poumon mwen rèd.
Poo-moh mwayh rehd.

My child / husband / wife is ill.
Pitit mwen / mari mwen / madanm mwen malad.
Pee-teet mwayh / mah-ree mwayh / mah-dahm mwayh mah-lahd.

He / she has a fever.
Li gen yon fyèv.
Lee gayh yohh feey-ehv.

I have _____

	Mwen gen _____.
	Mwayh gayh
diarrhea.	dyare
	dee-ah-ray
chest pain.	doulè nan lestomak.
	doo-leh nah
	lay-stoh-mahk
pain here.	doulè isi.
	doo-leh ee-see
a sore throat.	doulè nan gòj.
	doo-leh nah **gawj**
an earache.	doulè nan zorèy
	doo-leh nah **zoh-ray**
a headache	tèt fè mal
	teht feh **mahl**
a cough.	M'ap touse.
	Mah p' too-say
a cold.	Mwen gripe.
	Mwayh gree-pay

I've been vomiting.
Mwen te vomi.
Mwayh tay **voh-mee.**

How many times?
Konbyen fwa?
Kohh-bee-yehn fwah

After
apre
ahp-ray

How many days?
Konbyen jou?
Kohh-bee-yehn joo

Before
avan
Ah-vahh

Morning	**afternoon**	**at night**
Maten	*apremidi*	*lannwit*
Mah-tay	ah-pray-mee-dee	**lah-nweet**

After eating
Apre manje
Ah-pray mahn-jay

during
pandan
pahh-dahh

PATIENT INFORMATION

Write your name / your address.   signature
Ekri non ou / adrès ou.   *siyati*
__Ay__-kree **noh** oo / **ah**-drehs **oo.**   see-yah-tee

Write your phone number.
Ekri nimewo telefòn ou.
__Ay-kree__ nee-meh-woh **tay-lay-fohn** oo.

Write your date of birth.   **When were you born?**
Ekri dat ou fèt.   *Ki lè ou fèt?*
__Ay-kree__ daht **oo** feht.   **Kee leh oo feht?**

Write the name / phone number of your closest relative.
Ekri non ak nimewo telefòn moun ki pi pwòch ou.
__Ay__-kree **nohh** ahk **nee-**meh-**woh** moon **kee** pee **pwawsh** oo a.

Write the name of your employer.
Ekri non patwon ou.
__Ay-kree__ **nohh** pah-**twohn** oo.

Do you have a health insurance card?
Eske ou gen kat asirans pou sante ou?
__Ehs-keh__ oo **gayh** kaht **ah-see-rahns** poo **sahn-tay** oo?

Do you have a passport?
Eske ou gen yon paspò?
__Ehs__-keh **oo** gayh **yohh** pahs-**paw?**

Do you have an identification card?
Eske ou gen kat idantite?
__Ehs-keh__ oo **gehh** kaht **ee-dahn-tee-tay?**

I cannot read this. Write it again please.
Mwen pa kapab li sa. Fè ankò sivouple.
__Mwayh__ pah **kah-pahb** lee **sah.** Feh **ahng-kaw** see-voo-play.

Is your child ill?
Eske pitit ou a malad?
Ehs-keh **pee-teet** oo **ah** mah-lahd?

Does your child have a fever?
Eske pitit ou a gen lafyèv?
Ehs-keh **pee-teet** oo **ah** gayh **lah-feey-ehv?**

Has your child had vomiting / diarrhea?
Eske pitit ou a gen vomisman / dyare?
Ehs-keh **pee-teet** oo **ah** gayh **voh-mees-mah** / dee-ah-ray?

For how many days?
Depi konbyen jou?
Day-pee **kohh-beey-ehn** joo?

Has your child complained of pain?
Eske pitit ou konn plenn ak doulè?
Ehs-keh **pee-teet** oo kohn **playn** ahk **doo-leh?**

Has he/she received any immunizations?
Eske l' te pran vaksen?
Ehs-keh l' tay prahn vahk-sayh?

Do you know which vaccines? Do you have immunization card?
Eske ou konnen ki kalite vaksen? Eske ou gen kat vaksen?
Ehs-keh oo **koh-nay** kee **kah-lee-tay** / ehs-keh oo gayh **kaht vahk-sehh?**

Please hold your child while I give the injection.
Tanpri kenbe pitit la pandan m'ap ba li piki a.
Tahm-pree **kaym-bay** pee-teet **la** pah-dah **mahp** bah **lee pee-kee** ah.

Your child has an infection.
Pitit ou a gen yon enfeksyon.
Pee-teet oo **ah** gayh yohh **ayh-fayk-seey-ohh.**

Have this prescription filled.
Al ranpli preskripsyon sa a.
Ahl rahm-plee **pray-skreep-seey-ohh** sahh ah.

P
E
D
I
A
T
R
I
C
S

PROBLEM DRINKING

Do you drink alcohol every day?
Eske ou bwè klèren chak jou?
Ehs-keh oo bweh **kleh-rayh** shahk joo?

How many drinks each day?
Konbyen ou konsime pa jou?
koh-bee-yehn goh-day pah joo

How do you drink your alcohol, by the glass or bottle?
Kòman ou bwè alkòl ou, pa gode oubyen boutey?
Kaw-mahh oo **bweh** ahl-kawl **oo,** pah **goh-day** oo-bee-yehn **boo-tay?**

Do you often have six or more drinks in one day?
Eske ou toujou bwè 6 gode oubyen plis nan yon jou?
Ehs-keh oo **too-joo** bweh **sees** goh-day **oo-beey-ehn** plees **nah** yohh **joo?**

Do you ever feel the need to cut down on your drinking?
Eske ou pa janm santi ou bezwen redwi sa ou bwè?
Ehs-keh oo pah jahm **sahn-tee** oo **behz-wayh** ray-dwee **sah** oo **bweh?**

Do you ever feel guilty about drinking?
Eske ou santi ou wont lè ou bwè alkòl?
Ehs-keh oo **sahn-tee** oo **wohnt** leh **oo** bweh ahl-kawl?

Once or twice a week?
Youn oubyen de fwa pa semèn?
Yoon **oo-beey-ehn** day fwah pah **say-mehn?**

We have a program to help you stop drinking.
Nou gen yon pwogram ki ka ede ou sispan bwè alkòl.
Noo **gehh** yohh **pwoh-grahm** poo **noo** kah **ay-day** oo **sees-pahn** bweh.

Do you want to stop drinking?
Eske ou vle sispann bwè alkòl?
Ehs-keh oo **vlay** sees-pahn **bweh** ahl-kawl?

We will make an appointment for you.
Nou pral mete yon randevou pou ou.
Noo prahl **may-tay** yohh **rahn-day-voo** poo **ou.**

SEXUALLY TRANSMITTED DISEASES

Are you currently sexually active?
Eske ou fèk sòt kouche ak fi / gason?
Ehs-keh oo fehk sawt koo-shay ahk fee / gah-sohh?

Do you have more than one sex partner?
Eske ou gen pliske yon menaj?
Ehs-keh oo gayh plees-keh yohh may-nahj?

Is it painful to urinate?
Eske ou gen doulè lè ou pipi?
Ehs-keh oo gehh doo-leh leh oo pee-pee?

Do you have a vaginal discharge?
Eske ou ap fè dechay sòt nan vajin?
Ehs-keh oo ahp feh day-shahy-ee sawt nah vah-jeen?

We need to take a cervical specimen.
Nou dwe pran echantiyon po nan vajin.
Noo dway prahn ay-shahn-teey-ohn poh nah vah-jeen.

You have (don't have) a sexually transmitted disease.
Ou gen (pa gen) yon maladi kontamine seksyalman.
Oo gen (pa gen) yohh mah-lah-dee kohn-tah-mee-nay sayk-seey-ahl-mah.

You have clamydia / gonorrhea/ syphilis.
Ou gen klamidiya / grenn chalè / sifilis
<u>Oo</u> gayh <u>klah-mee-deey-ah</u> / grehn <u>shah-leh</u> /
see-fee-lees.

You only have a urinary infection. No other disease!
Pipi ou sèlman kontamine. Pa gen lòt maladi!
<u>Pee-pee</u> oo <u>sehl-mah</u> kohn-tahm-ee-neh, pa <u>gehh</u> lawt
mah-lah-<u>dee</u>!

Here is a prescription for antibiotics.
Sa se yon preskripsyon pou antibiyòtic.
<u>Sa</u> say <u>yohh</u> pray-skreep-seey-ohh <u>poo</u>
<u>ahn-tee-bee</u>-aw-teek.

Tell your sex partner(s) to visit the doctor.
Di menaj ou al wè doktè.
<u>Dee</u> may-<u>naj</u> oo <u>ahl</u> weh <u>dohk</u>-teh.

Do you ever have sores on your genitals?
Eske ou janm gen bouton nan pati jenital ou?
<u>Ehs-keh</u> oo <u>jahm</u> gayh <u>boo-tohh</u> nan <u>pah-tee</u>
jay-nee-tahl <u>ou?</u>

You may have the herpes virus.
Petèt ou ka gen viris hepèt.
<u>Pay-teht</u> oo <u>kah</u> gayh <u>vee-rees</u> hay-peht.

Are you pregnant?
Eske ou asent?
<u>Ehs-keh oo ah-saynt?</u>

SMALL TALK

Do you speak English?
Eske ou pale Anglè?
Ehs-keh oo **pah-lay** Ahng-gleh?

a little
toupiti
too-pee-tee

I do not speak Creole (English).
Mwen pa pale Kreyòl (Anglè).
Mwayh pah **pahl-ay** kray-awl (ahng-gleh).

Do you understand?
Eske ou konprann?
Ehs-keh oo **kohm-prahn?**

I don't understand.
Mwen pa konprann.
Mway pa **kohm-prahn**.

Have you been here before?
Eske ou konn vin isit la deja?
Ehs-keh oo **kohn** veen **ees-it** lah **day-jah?**

Do you have a husband / wife?
Eske ou gen mari / madanm?
Ehs-keh oo gayh **ma-ree** / mah-dahm?

Are you married?
Eske ou marye?
...**mah-ree-ay?**

Do you have children?
Eske ou gen pitit?
Ehs-keh oo gayh **pee-teet?**

Answer yes or no.
Reponn wi ou non.
Ray-pohn wee oo **noh**

Are you ill?
Eske ou malad?
Ehs-keh oo **mah-lahd?**

You don't need to be afraid. We'll take care of you.
Ou pa bezwen pè. N'ap pran swen ou.
Oo pa **behz-wayh** peh. Nahp **prahh sway**h oo.

TAKING VITALS

Undress and put on this gown, please.
Sivouple dezabiye, epi mete wòb sa.
See-voo-play, dayz-ah-bee-ay, ay-pee may-tay wob sa.

Sit down, please!
Chita, sivouple!
Shee-tah, see-voo-pleh.

Lie down.
Kouche.
Koo-shay.

I am going to take your temperature.
M'ap kontwole tanperati ou.
Mahp kohn-twohl-ay tahm-pay-rah-tee oo.

I am going to take your blood pressure.
M'ap kontwole tansyson ou.
Mahp kohn-twohl-ay tahn-seey-ohn oo.

We need to weigh you.
N'ap pran pwa ou.
Nahp prahh pwah oo.

Follow me.
Swiv mwen.
Sweev mwayh.

We need a urine sample / blood sample.
Nou bezwen pran pipi ou / san ou.
Noo behz-way prahh pee-pee oo / sahh oo.

Hold still!
Pa bouje!
Pah boo-jay!

Take off your sleeve.
Retire manch ou.
Ray-tee-ray mahhsh oo.

Put your arm here.
Mete bra ou isi.
May-tay brah oo ee-see.

Put on your clothes.
Abiye ou.
Ah-bee-ay oo.

clothes
rad
rahd

TB SCREENING & CHEST X-RAY

Have you been diagnosed with tuberculosis?
Eske ou pase maladi tibèkiloz deja?
Ehs-keh oo pah-say mah-lah-dee tee-beh-kee-lohz day-jah?

Do you smoke cigarettes?
Eske ou fimen sigarèt?
Ehs-keh oo fee-may see-gah-reht?

How many per day?
Konbyen pa jou?
Kohh-bee-yehn pa joo?

How many years have you smoked?
Konbyen lane ou te fimen?
Kohh-beey-ehn lah-nay oo tay fee-may?

Do you have a cough?
Eske ou gen tous?
Ehs-keh oo gayh toos?

Does it produce sputum?
Eske l' fè ou krache?
Ehs-keh l' fay oo krah-shay?

Is there blood in the sputum?
Eske ou wè san nan krache a?
Ehs-keh oo weh sahn nah krah-shay ah?

This is a skin test for tuberculosis.
Sa se yon egzamen po pou tibèkiloz.
Sah say yohh ayg-zahm-ay poh poo tee-beh-kee-lohz.

Very important!
Trèz enpòtan!
Trehz ayh-paw tahh!

Come back in three days for us to see the results.
Retounen nan twa jou pou nou ka wè rezilta a.
Ray-too-nay nah twah joo poo noo kah weh ray-zeel-tah ah.

TB SCREENING & CHEST X-RAY

You need to have a chest X-ray.
Ou bezwen yon radyografi.
<u>Oo behz-way</u>h yohh <u>rah-deey-oh-grah-fee.</u>

Please put on this apron.
Sivouple mete tabliye sa.
<u>See-voo-play</u> may-tay <u>tah-blee-ay</u> sah.

Stand facing the wall.
Kanpe, gade sou mi.
<u>Kahm-pay,</u> gah-day <u>soo</u> mee.

Put your chin here.
Mete manton isi.
<u>May-tay</u> mahn-tohh <u>ee-see.</u>

Don't move.
Pa souke kò ou.
<u>Pah</u> soo-kay <u>kaw</u> oo.

Roll your shoulders forward.
Koube epòl ou.
<u>Koo-bay</u> ay-pawl <u>oo.</u>

Take a deep breath and hold it.
Enspire fò epi kenbe l'.
<u>Ray-spee-ray</u> faw <u>eh-pee</u> kaym-bay <u>l'</u>

Relax!
Kalme.
<u>Kahl-may</u>

Turn sideways.
Vire lòt bò.
<u>Vee-ray</u> lawt <u>baw.</u>

That's all!
Sa sifi!.
Sah <u>see-fee!</u>

What caused the injury?
Kisa ki lakòz ou blese konsa?
Kee-sah kee lah-kawz oo blay-say kohn-sah?

Where does it hurt?
Ki kote l' fè ou mal?
Kee koh-tay l' feh oo mahl?

Does it hurt when I press here?
Eske l' fè ou mal lè m' peze la?
Ehs-kehl feh oo mahl lehm pay-zay lah?

You may have broken your arm / leg / rib / nose.
Petèt ou gen lè kase ponyèt ou / janm ou / zo kòt / nen.
Pay-teht oo gayh leh kah-say poh-yeht oo / jahm oo / zoh kawt / nay.

Do not move either your head or neck.
Pa vire ni tèt ou ni kou ou.
Pah vee-ray nee teht oo nee koo oo.

You (he/she) will need an X-ray.
Ou (li) ap bezwen yon radyografi.
Oo (lee) ahp behz-wayh yohh rah-deey-oh-grah-fee
It is only a sprain.
Se sèlman yon antòs / antòch.
Say sehl-mah yohh ahn-taws / ahn-tawsh.

I need to clean the wound. This may hurt a little.
M' bezwen netwaye blesi a. Li ka fè ou mal tou piti.
Mwayh behz-wayh nay-twah-yay blay-say ah. Lee kah feh oo mal too-pee-tee.

You will need stitches.
N'ap bezwen koud li.
Nahp behz-wayh kood lee.

When was your last tetanus shot?
Ki dènye fwa ou te pran piki pou tetanus?
Kee dehn-yay fwah oo tay prahn pee-kee poo tay-tah-noos?

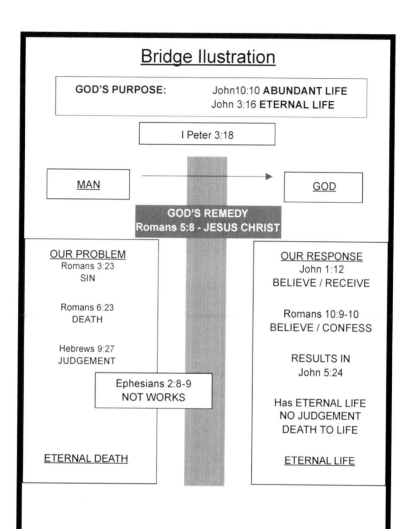

Bridge Ilustration

GOD'S PURPOSE: John10:10 **ABUNDANT LIFE**
John 3:16 **ETERNAL LIFE**

I Peter 3:18

MAN　　　　　　　　　　　　　　　GOD

**GOD'S REMEDY
Romans 5:8 - JESUS CHRIST**

OUR PROBLEM
Romans 3:23
SIN

Romans 6:23
DEATH

Hebrews 9:27
JUDGEMENT

Ephesians 2:8-9
NOT WORKS

ETERNAL DEATH

OUR RESPONSE
John 1:12
BELIEVE / RECEIVE

Romans 10:9-10
BELIEVE / CONFESS

RESULTS IN
John 5:24

Has ETERNAL LIFE
NO JUDGEMENT
DEATH TO LIFE

ETERNAL LIFE

Man constantly seeks a way to God. We don't have to create a new way. God has already made the way through His Son, Jesus Christ. We just have to obey God's plan. Repent and follow Jesus.

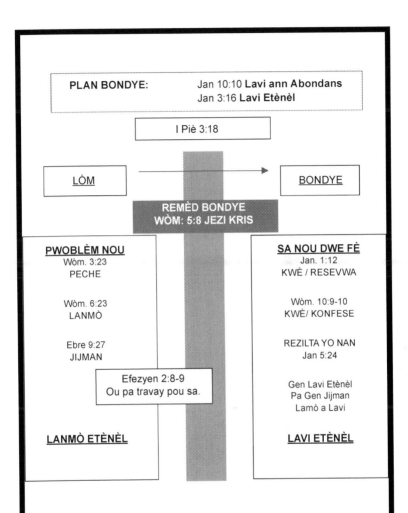

Lòm toujou ap chèche mwayen pou jwenn Bondye. Nou pa bezwen fè nouvo chemen. Bondye te deja fè mwayen atravè sèl pitit Li, Jezi Kris. Nou sèlman dwe obeyi plan Bondye epi mete tout konfyans nou nan Jezi Kris ki te peye dèt pou nou lè Li te mouri sou lakwa pou peche nou. Nou dwe repanti, vire do bay Satan epi swiv Jezi.

Printed in the United States
By Bookmasters